MACRO TRACKING JOURNAL

&

NUTRITION LOG BOOK

Log Period:

_____ to _____

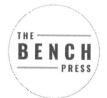

HOW TO USE THIS BOOK

A quick guide on getting the most from this daily macro tracker.

GETTING CLEAR ON YOUR MOTIVATION AND GOALS

At the start of this book you'll find space for writing your key drivers and motivators. Use these pages to understand why you want to achieve the goals you set. They'll be easier to hit when you can connect emotionally to your underlying 'why'.

Think about the top goals you want to achieve over the next two months. Is it to consistently stick to your macros each day? To gain or lose size in a certain area? To better manage food cravings? Note them all down in the goals section.

INITIAL & MONTHLY CHECK-IN

Record your starting measurements and monitor your progress with an additional check-in after one month.

DAILY FOOD LOGS WITH HEALTH INVENTORY

Record up to five meals a day with space for logging calories, protein, carbohydrates and fats. Total up your daily intakes at the bottom and note whether you're under or over target.

Use the corresponding health inventory to understand factors which could be helping or inhibiting your progress:

- Does the intensity of your training impact your food intake?

- What peri-workout nutrition strategy works for you? (Think pre-workout drinks/supplements, intra-workout boosters and post-workout meals/shakes)

- Are you feeling hungry today and what's your overall mood?

- Did you hit your daily water intake and are you well hydrated?

- What stage in your monthly cycle are you? Do you notice any particular food cravings at certain times of the month?

FINAL CHECK-IN

Record your final measurements and compare against your initial check-in to track physique progress over the period.

MOTIVATION & GOALS RE-CAP

Use these pages to reflect on your initial goals and note down achievements or reasons for not hitting your targets this time around.

WHAT IS MY WHY?

What is my motivation? What really drives me to reach my goals?

MACROS & NUTRITION GOALS

DAILY MACRONUTRIENT TARGETS

Calories:

Protein:

Carbohydrates:

Fats:

NUTRITION GOALS

Goal 1:

By when?   How?

Goal 2:

By when?   How?

Goal 3:

By when?   How?

HEALTHY LIVING GOALS

Goal 1:

By when?   How?

Goal 2:

By when?   How?

PHYSIQUE GOALS

Goal 1:

By when?   How?

Goal 2:

By when?   How?

NOTES

INITIAL CHECK-IN

DATE: /   /   DAY: M   T   W   T   F   S   S

Weight:

Body fat %:

Lean mass %:

Water %:

MEASUREMENTS

Neck:

Shoulders:

Chest / Bust:

Bicep (Left):   Bicep (Right):

Waist:

Hips:

Glutes:

Thigh (Left):   Thigh (Right):

Knee (Left):   Knee (Right):

Calf (Left):   Calf (Right):

NOTES

DATE: / /   DAY: M T W T F S S

HEALTH INVENTORY

TRAINING & IMPACT

Training day?:   ● HELL YEAH!   ● ACTIVE REST   ● DAY OFF

Intensity: ● HEAVY   ● AVERAGE   ● LIGHT

PERI-WORKOUT NUTRITION

Pre-workout:, intra- & post-workout nutrition / supplements:

MOOD & HUNGER

Hunger level?:   ● UNBEARABLE!   ● I CAN DEAL   ● WHAT HUNGER?

Overall mood:

CRAVINGS & TIME OF MONTH

Stage of menstrual cycle?:   ● MENSTRUAL   ● FOLLICULAR

Day: ● OVULATION   ● LUTEAL

Any cravings today?:

HYDRATION

Water intake: ● OVER TARGET!   ● ON TRACK   ● MUST DO BETTER

Glasses:

NOTES

DAILY FOOD LOG

MEAL 1 Time: _____	PROTEIN	CARBS	FATS	CALORIES

MEAL 2 Time: _____	PROTEIN	CARBS	FATS	CALORIES

MEAL 3 Time: _____	PROTEIN	CARBS	FATS	CALORIES

MEAL 4 Time: _____	PROTEIN	CARBS	FATS	CALORIES

MEAL 5 Time: _____	PROTEIN	CARBS	FATS	CALORIES

DAILY TOTALS:				
UNDER / OVER TARGET:				

DATE: / / DAY: M T W T F S S

HEALTH INVENTORY

TRAINING & IMPACT

Training day?: ● HELL YEAH! ● ACTIVE REST ● DAY OFF

Intensity: ● HEAVY ● AVERAGE ● LIGHT

PERI-WORKOUT NUTRITION

Pre-workout:, intra- & post-workout nutrition / supplements:

MOOD & HUNGER

Hunger level?: ● UNBEARABLE! ● I CAN DEAL ● WHAT HUNGER?

Overall mood:

CRAVINGS & TIME OF MONTH

Stage of menstrual cycle?: ● MENSTRUAL ● FOLLICULAR

Day: ● OVULATION ● LUTEAL

Any cravings today?:

HYDRATION

Water intake: ● OVER TARGET! ● ON TRACK ● MUST DO BETTER

Glasses:

NOTES

DAILY FOOD LOG

MEAL 1 Time: _____	PROTEIN	CARBS	FATS	CALORIES

MEAL 2 Time: _____	PROTEIN	CARBS	FATS	CALORIES

MEAL 3 Time: _____	PROTEIN	CARBS	FATS	CALORIES

MEAL 4 Time: _____	PROTEIN	CARBS	FATS	CALORIES

MEAL 5 Time: _____	PROTEIN	CARBS	FATS	CALORIES

DAILY TOTALS:				
UNDER / OVER TARGET:				

DATE: /   /   DAY: M   T   W   T   F   S   S

HEALTH INVENTORY

TRAINING & IMPACT

Training day?:   ● HELL YEAH!   ● ACTIVE REST   ● DAY OFF

Intensity: ● HEAVY   ● AVERAGE   ● LIGHT

PERI-WORKOUT NUTRITION

Pre-workout:, intra- & post-workout nutrition / supplements:

....

....

....

MOOD & HUNGER

Hunger level?:   ● UNBEARABLE!   ● I CAN DEAL   ● WHAT HUNGER?

Overall mood: ....

CRAVINGS & TIME OF MONTH

Stage of menstrual cycle?:   ● MENSTRUAL   ● FOLLICULAR

Day: ● OVULATION   ● LUTEAL

Any cravings today?: ....

HYDRATION

Water intake: ● OVER TARGET!   ● ON TRACK   ● MUST DO BETTER

Glasses: _____

NOTES

....

....

DAILY FOOD LOG

MEAL 1	Time: _____	PROTEIN	CARBS	FATS	CALORIES

MEAL 2	Time: _____	PROTEIN	CARBS	FATS	CALORIES

MEAL 3	Time: _____	PROTEIN	CARBS	FATS	CALORIES

MEAL 4	Time: _____	PROTEIN	CARBS	FATS	CALORIES

MEAL 5	Time: _____	PROTEIN	CARBS	FATS	CALORIES

	PROTEIN	CARBS	FATS
DAILY TOTALS:			
UNDER / OVER TARGET:			

DATE: /   /   DAY: M   T   W   T   F   S   S

HEALTH INVENTORY

TRAINING & IMPACT

Training day?:   ● HELL YEAH!   ● ACTIVE REST   ● DAY OFF

Intensity: ● HEAVY   ● AVERAGE   ● LIGHT

PERI-WORKOUT NUTRITION

Pre-workout:, intra- & post-workout nutrition / supplements:

MOOD & HUNGER

Hunger level?:   ● UNBEARABLE!   ● I CAN DEAL   ● WHAT HUNGER?

Overall mood:

CRAVINGS & TIME OF MONTH

Stage of menstrual cycle?:   ● MENSTRUAL   ● FOLLICULAR

Day: ● OVULATION   ● LUTEAL

Any cravings today?:

HYDRATION

Water intake: ● OVER TARGET!   ● ON TRACK   ● MUST DO BETTER

Glasses:

NOTES

DAILY FOOD LOG

MEAL 1 Time: _____	PROTEIN	CARBS	FATS	CALORIES

MEAL 2 Time: _____	PROTEIN	CARBS	FATS	CALORIES

MEAL 3 Time: _____	PROTEIN	CARBS	FATS	CALORIES

MEAL 4 Time: _____	PROTEIN	CARBS	FATS	CALORIES

MEAL 5 Time: _____	PROTEIN	CARBS	FATS	CALORIES

DAILY TOTALS:				
UNDER / OVER TARGET:				

DATE: /   /   DAY: M T W T F S S

HEALTH INVENTORY

TRAINING & IMPACT

Training day?:   ● HELL YEAH!   ● ACTIVE REST   ● DAY OFF
Intensity: ● HEAVY   ● AVERAGE   ● LIGHT

PERI-WORKOUT NUTRITION

Pre-workout:, intra- & post-workout nutrition / supplements:

_____

_____

_____

_____

MOOD & HUNGER

Hunger level?:   ● UNBEARABLE!   ● I CAN DEAL   ● WHAT HUNGER?
Overall mood: _____

CRAVINGS & TIME OF MONTH

Stage of menstrual cycle?:   ● MENSTRUAL   ● FOLLICULAR
Day: ● OVULATION   ● LUTEAL

Any cravings today?: _____

HYDRATION

Water intake: ● OVER TARGET!   ● ON TRACK   ● MUST DO BETTER
Glasses: _____

NOTES
_____

_____

_____

DAILY FOOD LOG

MEAL 1 Time: _____	PROTEIN	CARBS	FATS	CALORIES

MEAL 2 Time: _____	PROTEIN	CARBS	FATS	CALORIES

MEAL 3 Time: _____	PROTEIN	CARBS	FATS	CALORIES

MEAL 4 Time: _____	PROTEIN	CARBS	FATS	CALORIES

MEAL 5 Time: _____	PROTEIN	CARBS	FATS	CALORIES

DAILY TOTALS:				
UNDER / OVER TARGET:				

DATE: / /   DAY: M T W T F S S

HEALTH INVENTORY

TRAINING & IMPACT

Training day?:   ⬤ HELL YEAH!   ⬤ ACTIVE REST   ⬤ DAY OFF
Intensity: ⬤ HEAVY   ⬤ AVERAGE   ⬤ LIGHT

PERI-WORKOUT NUTRITION

Pre-workout:, intra- & post-workout nutrition / supplements:

MOOD & HUNGER

Hunger level?:   ⬤ UNBEARABLE!   ⬤ I CAN DEAL   ⬤ WHAT HUNGER?
Overall mood:

CRAVINGS & TIME OF MONTH

Stage of menstrual cycle?:   ⬤ MENSTRUAL   ⬤ FOLLICULAR
Day: ⬤ OVULATION   ⬤ LUTEAL

Any cravings today?:

HYDRATION

Water intake: ⬤ OVER TARGET!   ⬤ ON TRACK   ⬤ MUST DO BETTER
Glasses:

NOTES

DAILY FOOD LOG

MEAL 1 Time: _____	PROTEIN	CARBS	FATS	CALORIES

MEAL 2 Time: _____	PROTEIN	CARBS	FATS	CALORIES

MEAL 3 Time: _____	PROTEIN	CARBS	FATS	CALORIES

MEAL 4 Time: _____	PROTEIN	CARBS	FATS	CALORIES

MEAL 5 Time: _____	PROTEIN	CARBS	FATS	CALORIES

	PROTEIN	CARBS	FATS	CALORIES
DAILY TOTALS:				
UNDER / OVER TARGET:				

DATE: / / DAY: M T W T F S S

HEALTH INVENTORY

TRAINING & IMPACT

Training day?: ● HELL YEAH! ● ACTIVE REST ● DAY OFF

Intensity: ● HEAVY ● AVERAGE ● LIGHT

PERI-WORKOUT NUTRITION

Pre-workout:, intra- & post-workout nutrition / supplements:

MOOD & HUNGER

Hunger level?: ● UNBEARABLE! ● I CAN DEAL ● WHAT HUNGER?

Overall mood:

CRAVINGS & TIME OF MONTH

Stage of menstrual cycle?: ● MENSTRUAL ● FOLLICULAR

Day: ● OVULATION ● LUTEAL

Any cravings today?:

HYDRATION

Water intake: ● OVER TARGET! ● ON TRACK ● MUST DO BETTER

Glasses:

NOTES

DAILY FOOD LOG

MEAL 1 Time: _____	PROTEIN	CARBS	FATS	CALORIES

MEAL 2 Time: _____	PROTEIN	CARBS	FATS	CALORIES

MEAL 3 Time: _____	PROTEIN	CARBS	FATS	CALORIES

MEAL 4 Time: _____	PROTEIN	CARBS	FATS	CALORIES

MEAL 5 Time: _____	PROTEIN	CARBS	FATS	CALORIES

DAILY TOTALS:				
UNDER / OVER TARGET:				

DATE: / / DAY: M T W T F S S

HEALTH INVENTORY

TRAINING & IMPACT

Training day?: ● HELL YEAH! ● ACTIVE REST ● DAY OFF
Intensity: ● HEAVY ● AVERAGE ● LIGHT

PERI-WORKOUT NUTRITION

Pre-workout:, intra- & post-workout nutrition / supplements:

MOOD & HUNGER

Hunger level?: ● UNBEARABLE! ● I CAN DEAL ● WHAT HUNGER?
Overall mood:

CRAVINGS & TIME OF MONTH

Stage of menstrual cycle?: ● MENSTRUAL ● FOLLICULAR
Day: ● OVULATION ● LUTEAL

Any cravings today?:

HYDRATION

Water intake: ● OVER TARGET! ● ON TRACK ● MUST DO BETTER
Glasses:

NOTES

DAILY FOOD LOG

MEAL 1 Time: _____	PROTEIN	CARBS	FATS	CALORIES

MEAL 2 Time: _____	PROTEIN	CARBS	FATS	CALORIES

MEAL 3 Time: _____	PROTEIN	CARBS	FATS	CALORIES

MEAL 4 Time: _____	PROTEIN	CARBS	FATS	CALORIES

MEAL 5 Time: _____	PROTEIN	CARBS	FATS	CALORIES

DAILY TOTALS:				
UNDER / OVER TARGET:				

DATE: /   /   DAY: M   T   W   T   F   S   S

HEALTH INVENTORY

TRAINING & IMPACT

Training day?:   ⬤ HELL YEAH!   ⬤ ACTIVE REST   ⬤ DAY OFF
Intensity: ⬤ HEAVY   ⬤ AVERAGE   ⬤ LIGHT

PERI-WORKOUT NUTRITION

Pre-workout:, intra- & post-workout nutrition / supplements:

MOOD & HUNGER

Hunger level?:   ⬤ UNBEARABLE!   ⬤ I CAN DEAL   ⬤ WHAT HUNGER?
Overall mood:

CRAVINGS & TIME OF MONTH

Stage of menstrual cycle?:   ⬤ MENSTRUAL   ⬤ FOLLICULAR
Day: ⬤ OVULATION   ⬤ LUTEAL

Any cravings today?:

HYDRATION

Water intake: ⬤ OVER TARGET!   ⬤ ON TRACK   ⬤ MUST DO BETTER
Glasses:

NOTES

DAILY FOOD LOG

MEAL 1 Time: _____	PROTEIN	CARBS	FATS	CALORIES

MEAL 2 Time: _____	PROTEIN	CARBS	FATS	CALORIES

MEAL 3 Time: _____	PROTEIN	CARBS	FATS	CALORIES

MEAL 4 Time: _____	PROTEIN	CARBS	FATS	CALORIES

MEAL 5 Time: _____	PROTEIN	CARBS	FATS	CALORIES

DAILY TOTALS:				
UNDER / OVER TARGET:				

DATE: /   /   DAY: M T W T F S S

HEALTH INVENTORY

TRAINING & IMPACT

Training day?:   ● HELL YEAH!   ● ACTIVE REST   ● DAY OFF

Intensity: ● HEAVY   ● AVERAGE   ● LIGHT

PERI-WORKOUT NUTRITION

Pre-workout:, intra- & post-workout nutrition / supplements:

....

....

....

MOOD & HUNGER

Hunger level?:   ● UNBEARABLE!   ● I CAN DEAL   ● WHAT HUNGER?

Overall mood: ....

CRAVINGS & TIME OF MONTH

Stage of menstrual cycle?:   ● MENSTRUAL   ● FOLLICULAR

Day: ● OVULATION   ● LUTEAL

Any cravings today?: ....

HYDRATION

Water intake: ● OVER TARGET!   ● ON TRACK   ● MUST DO BETTER

Glasses: ....

NOTES
....

....

DAILY FOOD LOG

MEAL 1 Time: _____	PROTEIN	CARBS	FATS	CALORIES

MEAL 2 Time: _____	PROTEIN	CARBS	FATS	CALORIES

MEAL 3 Time: _____	PROTEIN	CARBS	FATS	CALORIES

MEAL 4 Time: _____	PROTEIN	CARBS	FATS	CALORIES

MEAL 5 Time: _____	PROTEIN	CARBS	FATS	CALORIES

DAILY TOTALS:			
UNDER / OVER TARGET:			

DATE: / / DAY: M T W T F S S

HEALTH INVENTORY

TRAINING & IMPACT

Training day?: ⬤ HELL YEAH! ⬤ ACTIVE REST ⬤ DAY OFF

Intensity: ⬤ HEAVY ⬤ AVERAGE ⬤ LIGHT

PERI-WORKOUT NUTRITION

Pre-workout:, intra- & post-workout nutrition / supplements:

MOOD & HUNGER

Hunger level?: ⬤ UNBEARABLE! ⬤ I CAN DEAL ⬤ WHAT HUNGER?

Overall mood:

CRAVINGS & TIME OF MONTH

Stage of menstrual cycle?: ⬤ MENSTRUAL ⬤ FOLLICULAR

Day: ⬤ OVULATION ⬤ LUTEAL

Any cravings today?:

HYDRATION

Water intake: ⬤ OVER TARGET! ⬤ ON TRACK ⬤ MUST DO BETTER

Glasses:

NOTES

DAILY FOOD LOG

MEAL 1 Time: _____	PROTEIN	CARBS	FATS	CALORIES

MEAL 2 Time: _____	PROTEIN	CARBS	FATS	CALORIES

MEAL 3 Time: _____	PROTEIN	CARBS	FATS	CALORIES

MEAL 4 Time: _____	PROTEIN	CARBS	FATS	CALORIES

MEAL 5 Time: _____	PROTEIN	CARBS	FATS	CALORIES

DAILY TOTALS:			
UNDER / OVER TARGET:			

DATE: /   /   DAY: M T W T F S S

HEALTH INVENTORY

TRAINING & IMPACT

Training day?:   ● HELL YEAH!   ● ACTIVE REST   ● DAY OFF

Intensity: ● HEAVY   ● AVERAGE   ● LIGHT

PERI-WORKOUT NUTRITION

Pre-workout:, intra- & post-workout nutrition / supplements:

MOOD & HUNGER

Hunger level?:   ● UNBEARABLE!   ● I CAN DEAL   ● WHAT HUNGER?

Overall mood:

CRAVINGS & TIME OF MONTH

Stage of menstrual cycle?:   ● MENSTRUAL   ● FOLLICULAR

Day: ● OVULATION   ● LUTEAL

Any cravings today?:

HYDRATION

Water intake: ● OVER TARGET!   ● ON TRACK   ● MUST DO BETTER

Glasses:

NOTES

DAILY FOOD LOG

MEAL 1 Time: _____	PROTEIN	CARBS	FATS	CALORIES

MEAL 2 Time: _____	PROTEIN	CARBS	FATS	CALORIES

MEAL 3 Time: _____	PROTEIN	CARBS	FATS	CALORIES

MEAL 4 Time: _____	PROTEIN	CARBS	FATS	CALORIES

MEAL 5 Time: _____	PROTEIN	CARBS	FATS	CALORIES

DAILY TOTALS:				
UNDER / OVER TARGET:				

DATE: /   /   DAY: M   T   W   T   F   S   S

HEALTH INVENTORY

TRAINING & IMPACT

Training day?:   ● HELL YEAH!   ● ACTIVE REST   ● DAY OFF
Intensity: ● HEAVY   ● AVERAGE   ● LIGHT

PERI-WORKOUT NUTRITION

Pre-workout:, intra- & post-workout nutrition / supplements:

....

....

....

....

MOOD & HUNGER

Hunger level?:   ● UNBEARABLE!   ● I CAN DEAL   ● WHAT HUNGER?
Overall mood: ....

CRAVINGS & TIME OF MONTH

Stage of menstrual cycle?:   ● MENSTRUAL   ● FOLLICULAR
Day: ● OVULATION   ● LUTEAL

Any cravings today?: ....

HYDRATION

Water intake: ● OVER TARGET!   ● ON TRACK   ● MUST DO BETTER
Glasses: ....

NOTES
....

....

....

DAILY FOOD LOG

MEAL 1 Time: ___	PROTEIN	CARBS	FATS	CALORIES

MEAL 2 Time: ___	PROTEIN	CARBS	FATS	CALORIES

MEAL 3 Time: ___	PROTEIN	CARBS	FATS	CALORIES

MEAL 4 Time: ___	PROTEIN	CARBS	FATS	CALORIES

MEAL 5 Time: ___	PROTEIN	CARBS	FATS	CALORIES

	PROTEIN	CARBS	FATS	CALORIES
DAILY TOTALS:				
UNDER / OVER TARGET:				

DATE: /   /   DAY: M T W T F S S

HEALTH INVENTORY

TRAINING & IMPACT

Training day?:   ● HELL YEAH!   ● ACTIVE REST   ● DAY OFF

Intensity: ● HEAVY   ● AVERAGE   ● LIGHT

PERI-WORKOUT NUTRITION

Pre-workout:, intra- & post-workout nutrition / supplements:

MOOD & HUNGER

Hunger level?:   ● UNBEARABLE!   ● I CAN DEAL   ● WHAT HUNGER?

Overall mood:

CRAVINGS & TIME OF MONTH

Stage of menstrual cycle?:   ● MENSTRUAL   ● FOLLICULAR

Day: ● OVULATION   ● LUTEAL

Any cravings today?:

HYDRATION

Water intake: ● OVER TARGET!   ● ON TRACK   ● MUST DO BETTER

Glasses:

NOTES

DAILY FOOD LOG

MEAL 1	Time: _____	PROTEIN	CARBS	FATS	CALORIES

MEAL 2	Time: _____	PROTEIN	CARBS	FATS	CALORIES

MEAL 3	Time: _____	PROTEIN	CARBS	FATS	CALORIES

MEAL 4	Time: _____	PROTEIN	CARBS	FATS	CALORIES

MEAL 5	Time: _____	PROTEIN	CARBS	FATS	CALORIES

	PROTEIN	CARBS	FATS	CALORIES
DAILY TOTALS:				
UNDER / OVER TARGET:				

DATE: / / DAY: M T W T F S S

HEALTH INVENTORY

TRAINING & IMPACT

Training day?: ● HELL YEAH! ● ACTIVE REST ● DAY OFF

Intensity: ● HEAVY ● AVERAGE ● LIGHT

PERI-WORKOUT NUTRITION

Pre-workout:, intra- & post-workout nutrition / supplements:

....

....

....

MOOD & HUNGER

Hunger level?: ● UNBEARABLE! ● I CAN DEAL ● WHAT HUNGER?

Overall mood: ....

CRAVINGS & TIME OF MONTH

Stage of menstrual cycle?: ● MENSTRUAL ● FOLLICULAR

Day: ● OVULATION ● LUTEAL

Any cravings today?: ....

HYDRATION

Water intake: ● OVER TARGET! ● ON TRACK ● MUST DO BETTER

Glasses: ....

NOTES
....
....

DAILY FOOD LOG

MEAL 1	Time: _____	PROTEIN	CARBS	FATS	CALORIES

MEAL 2	Time: _____	PROTEIN	CARBS	FATS	CALORIES

MEAL 3	Time: _____	PROTEIN	CARBS	FATS	CALORIES

MEAL 4	Time: _____	PROTEIN	CARBS	FATS	CALORIES

MEAL 5	Time: _____	PROTEIN	CARBS	FATS	CALORIES

	PROTEIN	CARBS	FATS	CALORIES
DAILY TOTALS:				
UNDER / OVER TARGET:				

DATE: / / DAY: M T W T F S S

HEALTH INVENTORY

TRAINING & IMPACT

Training day?: ● HELL YEAH! ● ACTIVE REST ● DAY OFF
Intensity: ● HEAVY ● AVERAGE ● LIGHT

PERI-WORKOUT NUTRITION

Pre-workout:, intra- & post-workout nutrition / supplements:

MOOD & HUNGER

Hunger level?: ● UNBEARABLE! ● I CAN DEAL ● WHAT HUNGER?
Overall mood:

CRAVINGS & TIME OF MONTH

Stage of menstrual cycle?: ● MENSTRUAL ● FOLLICULAR
Day: ● OVULATION ● LUTEAL

Any cravings today?:

HYDRATION

Water intake: ● OVER TARGET! ● ON TRACK ● MUST DO BETTER
Glasses:

NOTES

DAILY FOOD LOG

MEAL 1	Time: _____	PROTEIN	CARBS	FATS	CALORIES

MEAL 2	Time: _____	PROTEIN	CARBS	FATS	CALORIES

MEAL 3	Time: _____	PROTEIN	CARBS	FATS	CALORIES

MEAL 4	Time: _____	PROTEIN	CARBS	FATS	CALORIES

MEAL 5	Time: _____	PROTEIN	CARBS	FATS	CALORIES

	PROTEIN	CARBS	FATS	CALORIES
DAILY TOTALS:				
UNDER / OVER TARGET:				

DATE: /   /   DAY: M T W T F S S

HEALTH INVENTORY

TRAINING & IMPACT

Training day?:   ● HELL YEAH!   ● ACTIVE REST   ● DAY OFF
Intensity: ● HEAVY   ● AVERAGE   ● LIGHT

PERI-WORKOUT NUTRITION

Pre-workout:, intra- & post-workout nutrition / supplements:

MOOD & HUNGER

Hunger level?:   ● UNBEARABLE!   ● I CAN DEAL   ● WHAT HUNGER?
Overall mood:

CRAVINGS & TIME OF MONTH

Stage of menstrual cycle?:   ● MENSTRUAL   ● FOLLICULAR
Day: ● OVULATION   ● LUTEAL

Any cravings today?:

HYDRATION

Water intake: ● OVER TARGET!   ● ON TRACK   ● MUST DO BETTER
Glasses:

NOTES

DAILY FOOD LOG

MEAL 1 Time: _____	PROTEIN	CARBS	FATS	CALORIES

MEAL 2 Time: _____	PROTEIN	CARBS	FATS	CALORIES

MEAL 3 Time: _____	PROTEIN	CARBS	FATS	CALORIES

MEAL 4 Time: _____	PROTEIN	CARBS	FATS	CALORIES

MEAL 5 Time: _____	PROTEIN	CARBS	FATS	CALORIES

	PROTEIN	CARBS	FATS	CALORIES
DAILY TOTALS:				
UNDER / OVER TARGET:				

DATE: /   /   DAY: M T W T F S S

HEALTH INVENTORY

TRAINING & IMPACT

Training day?:   ⬤ HELL YEAH!   ⬤ ACTIVE REST   ⬤ DAY OFF

Intensity: ⬤ HEAVY   ⬤ AVERAGE   ⬤ LIGHT

PERI-WORKOUT NUTRITION

Pre-workout:, intra- & post-workout nutrition / supplements:

MOOD & HUNGER

Hunger level?:   ⬤ UNBEARABLE!   ⬤ I CAN DEAL   ⬤ WHAT HUNGER?

Overall mood:

CRAVINGS & TIME OF MONTH

Stage of menstrual cycle?:   ⬤ MENSTRUAL   ⬤ FOLLICULAR

Day: ⬤ OVULATION   ⬤ LUTEAL

Any cravings today?:

HYDRATION

Water intake: ⬤ OVER TARGET!   ⬤ ON TRACK   ⬤ MUST DO BETTER

Glasses:

NOTES

DAILY FOOD LOG

MEAL 1 Time: _____	PROTEIN	CARBS	FATS	CALORIES

MEAL 2 Time: _____	PROTEIN	CARBS	FATS	CALORIES

MEAL 3 Time: _____	PROTEIN	CARBS	FATS	CALORIES

MEAL 4 Time: _____	PROTEIN	CARBS	FATS	CALORIES

MEAL 5 Time: _____	PROTEIN	CARBS	FATS	CALORIES

DAILY TOTALS:			
UNDER / OVER TARGET:			

DATE: / / DAY: M T W T F S S

HEALTH INVENTORY

TRAINING & IMPACT

Training day?: ● HELL YEAH! ● ACTIVE REST ● DAY OFF

Intensity: ● HEAVY ● AVERAGE ● LIGHT

PERI-WORKOUT NUTRITION

Pre-workout:, intra- & post-workout nutrition / supplements:

MOOD & HUNGER

Hunger level?: ● UNBEARABLE! ● I CAN DEAL ● WHAT HUNGER?

Overall mood:

CRAVINGS & TIME OF MONTH

Stage of menstrual cycle?: ● MENSTRUAL ● FOLLICULAR

Day: ● OVULATION ● LUTEAL

Any cravings today?:

HYDRATION

Water intake: ● OVER TARGET! ● ON TRACK ● MUST DO BETTER

Glasses:

NOTES

DAILY FOOD LOG

MEAL 1 Time: _____	PROTEIN	CARBS	FATS	CALORIES

MEAL 2 Time: _____	PROTEIN	CARBS	FATS	CALORIES

MEAL 3 Time: _____	PROTEIN	CARBS	FATS	CALORIES

MEAL 4 Time: _____	PROTEIN	CARBS	FATS	CALORIES

MEAL 5 Time: _____	PROTEIN	CARBS	FATS	CALORIES

	PROTEIN	CARBS	FATS	CALORIES
DAILY TOTALS:				
UNDER / OVER TARGET:				

DATE: / / DAY: M T W T F S S

HEALTH INVENTORY

TRAINING & IMPACT

Training day?: ● HELL YEAH! ● ACTIVE REST ● DAY OFF

Intensity: ● HEAVY ● AVERAGE ● LIGHT

PERI-WORKOUT NUTRITION

Pre-workout:, intra- & post-workout nutrition / supplements:

MOOD & HUNGER

Hunger level?: ● UNBEARABLE! ● I CAN DEAL ● WHAT HUNGER?

Overall mood:

CRAVINGS & TIME OF MONTH

Stage of menstrual cycle?: ● MENSTRUAL ● FOLLICULAR

Day: ● OVULATION ● LUTEAL

Any cravings today?:

HYDRATION

Water intake: ● OVER TARGET! ● ON TRACK ● MUST DO BETTER

Glasses:

NOTES

DAILY FOOD LOG

MEAL 1	Time: _____	PROTEIN	CARBS	FATS	CALORIES

MEAL 2	Time: _____	PROTEIN	CARBS	FATS	CALORIES

MEAL 3	Time: _____	PROTEIN	CARBS	FATS	CALORIES

MEAL 4	Time: _____	PROTEIN	CARBS	FATS	CALORIES

MEAL 5	Time: _____	PROTEIN	CARBS	FATS	CALORIES

DAILY TOTALS:

UNDER / OVER TARGET:

DATE: /   /   DAY: M   T   W   T   F   S   S

HEALTH INVENTORY

TRAINING & IMPACT

Training day?:   ● HELL YEAH!   ● ACTIVE REST   ● DAY OFF
Intensity: ● HEAVY   ● AVERAGE   ● LIGHT

PERI-WORKOUT NUTRITION

Pre-workout:, intra- & post-workout nutrition / supplements:

MOOD & HUNGER

Hunger level?:   ● UNBEARABLE!   ● I CAN DEAL   ● WHAT HUNGER?
Overall mood:

CRAVINGS & TIME OF MONTH

Stage of menstrual cycle?:   ● MENSTRUAL   ● FOLLICULAR
Day: ● OVULATION   ● LUTEAL

Any cravings today?:

HYDRATION

Water intake: ● OVER TARGET!   ● ON TRACK   ● MUST DO BETTER
Glasses:

NOTES

DAILY FOOD LOG

MEAL 1 Time: _____	PROTEIN	CARBS	FATS	CALORIES

MEAL 2 Time: _____	PROTEIN	CARBS	FATS	CALORIES

MEAL 3 Time: _____	PROTEIN	CARBS	FATS	CALORIES

MEAL 4 Time: _____	PROTEIN	CARBS	FATS	CALORIES

MEAL 5 Time: _____	PROTEIN	CARBS	FATS	CALORIES

	PROTEIN	CARBS	FATS	CALORIES
DAILY TOTALS:				
UNDER / OVER TARGET:				

DATE: /   /   DAY: M   T   W   T   F   S   S

HEALTH INVENTORY

TRAINING & IMPACT

Training day?:   ⬤ HELL YEAH!   ⬤ ACTIVE REST   ⬤ DAY OFF

Intensity: ⬤ HEAVY   ⬤ AVERAGE   ⬤ LIGHT

PERI-WORKOUT NUTRITION

Pre-workout:, intra- & post-workout nutrition / supplements:

MOOD & HUNGER

Hunger level?:   ⬤ UNBEARABLE!   ⬤ I CAN DEAL   ⬤ WHAT HUNGER?

Overall mood:

CRAVINGS & TIME OF MONTH

Stage of menstrual cycle?:   ⬤ MENSTRUAL   ⬤ FOLLICULAR

Day: ⬤ OVULATION   ⬤ LUTEAL

Any cravings today?:

HYDRATION

Water intake: ⬤ OVER TARGET!   ⬤ ON TRACK   ⬤ MUST DO BETTER

Glasses:

NOTES

DAILY FOOD LOG

MEAL 1 Time: _____	PROTEIN	CARBS	FATS	CALORIES

MEAL 2 Time: _____	PROTEIN	CARBS	FATS	CALORIES

MEAL 3 Time: _____	PROTEIN	CARBS	FATS	CALORIES

MEAL 4 Time: _____	PROTEIN	CARBS	FATS	CALORIES

MEAL 5 Time: _____	PROTEIN	CARBS	FATS	CALORIES

DAILY TOTALS:				
UNDER / OVER TARGET:				

DATE: / / DAY: M T W T F S S

HEALTH INVENTORY

TRAINING & IMPACT

Training day?: ● HELL YEAH! ● ACTIVE REST ● DAY OFF

Intensity: ● HEAVY ● AVERAGE ● LIGHT

PERI-WORKOUT NUTRITION

Pre-workout:, intra- & post-workout nutrition / supplements:

....

....

....

MOOD & HUNGER

Hunger level?: ● UNBEARABLE! ● I CAN DEAL ● WHAT HUNGER?

Overall mood: ....

CRAVINGS & TIME OF MONTH

Stage of menstrual cycle?: ● MENSTRUAL ● FOLLICULAR

Day: ● OVULATION ● LUTEAL

Any cravings today?: ....

HYDRATION

Water intake: ● OVER TARGET! ● ON TRACK ● MUST DO BETTER

Glasses: ....

NOTES
....
....

DAILY FOOD LOG

MEAL 1 Time: _____	PROTEIN	CARBS	FATS	CALORIES

MEAL 2 Time: _____	PROTEIN	CARBS	FATS	CALORIES

MEAL 3 Time: _____	PROTEIN	CARBS	FATS	CALORIES

MEAL 4 Time: _____	PROTEIN	CARBS	FATS	CALORIES

MEAL 5 Time: _____	PROTEIN	CARBS	FATS	CALORIES

DAILY TOTALS:				
UNDER / OVER TARGET:				

DATE: /   /   DAY: M   T   W   T   F   S   S

HEALTH INVENTORY

TRAINING & IMPACT

Training day?:   ⬤ HELL YEAH!   ⬤ ACTIVE REST   ⬤ DAY OFF

Intensity: ⬤ HEAVY   ⬤ AVERAGE   ⬤ LIGHT

PERI-WORKOUT NUTRITION

Pre-workout:, intra- & post-workout nutrition / supplements:

MOOD & HUNGER

Hunger level?:   ⬤ UNBEARABLE!   ⬤ I CAN DEAL   ⬤ WHAT HUNGER?

Overall mood:

CRAVINGS & TIME OF MONTH

Stage of menstrual cycle?:   ⬤ MENSTRUAL   ⬤ FOLLICULAR

Day: ⬤ OVULATION   ⬤ LUTEAL

Any cravings today?:

HYDRATION

Water intake: ⬤ OVER TARGET!   ⬤ ON TRACK   ⬤ MUST DO BETTER

Glasses:

NOTES

DAILY FOOD LOG

MEAL 1 Time: _____	PROTEIN	CARBS	FATS	CALORIES

MEAL 2 Time: _____	PROTEIN	CARBS	FATS	CALORIES

MEAL 3 Time: _____	PROTEIN	CARBS	FATS	CALORIES

MEAL 4 Time: _____	PROTEIN	CARBS	FATS	CALORIES

MEAL 5 Time: _____	PROTEIN	CARBS	FATS	CALORIES

DAILY TOTALS:				
UNDER / OVER TARGET:				

DATE: / / DAY: M T W T F S S

HEALTH INVENTORY

TRAINING & IMPACT

Training day?: ● HELL YEAH! ● ACTIVE REST ● DAY OFF

Intensity: ● HEAVY ● AVERAGE ● LIGHT

PERI-WORKOUT NUTRITION

Pre-workout:, intra- & post-workout nutrition / supplements:

MOOD & HUNGER

Hunger level?: ● UNBEARABLE! ● I CAN DEAL ● WHAT HUNGER?

Overall mood:

CRAVINGS & TIME OF MONTH

Stage of menstrual cycle?: ● MENSTRUAL ● FOLLICULAR

Day: ● OVULATION ● LUTEAL

Any cravings today?:

HYDRATION

Water intake: ● OVER TARGET! ● ON TRACK ● MUST DO BETTER

Glasses:

NOTES

DAILY FOOD LOG

MEAL 1	Time: _____	PROTEIN	CARBS	FATS	CALORIES

MEAL 2	Time: _____	PROTEIN	CARBS	FATS	CALORIES

MEAL 3	Time: _____	PROTEIN	CARBS	FATS	CALORIES

MEAL 4	Time: _____	PROTEIN	CARBS	FATS	CALORIES

MEAL 5	Time: _____	PROTEIN	CARBS	FATS	CALORIES

DAILY TOTALS:				
UNDER / OVER TARGET:				

DATE: / / DAY: M T W T F S S

HEALTH INVENTORY

TRAINING & IMPACT

Training day?: ● HELL YEAH! ● ACTIVE REST ● DAY OFF

Intensity: ● HEAVY ● AVERAGE ● LIGHT

PERI-WORKOUT NUTRITION

Pre-workout:, intra- & post-workout nutrition / supplements:

MOOD & HUNGER

Hunger level?: ● UNBEARABLE! ● I CAN DEAL ● WHAT HUNGER?

Overall mood:

CRAVINGS & TIME OF MONTH

Stage of menstrual cycle?: ● MENSTRUAL ● FOLLICULAR

Day: ● OVULATION ● LUTEAL

Any cravings today?:

HYDRATION

Water intake: ● OVER TARGET! ● ON TRACK ● MUST DO BETTER

Glasses:

NOTES

DAILY FOOD LOG

MEAL 1 Time: _____	PROTEIN	CARBS	FATS	CALORIES

MEAL 2 Time: _____	PROTEIN	CARBS	FATS	CALORIES

MEAL 3 Time: _____	PROTEIN	CARBS	FATS	CALORIES

MEAL 4 Time: _____	PROTEIN	CARBS	FATS	CALORIES

MEAL 5 Time: _____	PROTEIN	CARBS	FATS	CALORIES

	PROTEIN	CARBS	FATS	CALORIES
DAILY TOTALS:				
UNDER / OVER TARGET:				

DATE: / / DAY: M T W T F S S

HEALTH INVENTORY

TRAINING & IMPACT

Training day?: ● HELL YEAH! ● ACTIVE REST ● DAY OFF

Intensity: ● HEAVY ● AVERAGE ● LIGHT

PERI-WORKOUT NUTRITION

Pre-workout:, intra- & post-workout nutrition / supplements:

....

....

....

MOOD & HUNGER

Hunger level?: ● UNBEARABLE! ● I CAN DEAL ● WHAT HUNGER?

Overall mood: ....

CRAVINGS & TIME OF MONTH

Stage of menstrual cycle?: ● MENSTRUAL ● FOLLICULAR

Day: ● OVULATION ● LUTEAL

Any cravings today?: ....

HYDRATION

Water intake: ● OVER TARGET! ● ON TRACK ● MUST DO BETTER

Glasses: _____

NOTES
....
....

DAILY FOOD LOG

MEAL 1	Time: _____	PROTEIN	CARBS	FATS	CALORIES

MEAL 2	Time: _____	PROTEIN	CARBS	FATS	CALORIES

MEAL 3	Time: _____	PROTEIN	CARBS	FATS	CALORIES

MEAL 4	Time: _____	PROTEIN	CARBS	FATS	CALORIES

MEAL 5	Time: _____	PROTEIN	CARBS	FATS	CALORIES

DAILY TOTALS:				
UNDER / OVER TARGET:				

DATE: /   /   DAY: M T W T F S S

HEALTH INVENTORY

TRAINING & IMPACT

Training day?:   ● HELL YEAH!   ● ACTIVE REST   ● DAY OFF
Intensity: ● HEAVY   ● AVERAGE   ● LIGHT

PERI-WORKOUT NUTRITION

Pre-workout:, intra- & post-workout nutrition / supplements:

MOOD & HUNGER

Hunger level?:   ● UNBEARABLE!   ● I CAN DEAL   ● WHAT HUNGER?
Overall mood:

CRAVINGS & TIME OF MONTH

Stage of menstrual cycle?:   ● MENSTRUAL   ● FOLLICULAR
Day: ● OVULATION   ● LUTEAL

Any cravings today?:

HYDRATION

Water intake: ● OVER TARGET!   ● ON TRACK   ● MUST DO BETTER
Glasses:

NOTES

DAILY FOOD LOG

MEAL 1 Time: _____	PROTEIN	CARBS	FATS	CALORIES

MEAL 2 Time: _____	PROTEIN	CARBS	FATS	CALORIES

MEAL 3 Time: _____	PROTEIN	CARBS	FATS	CALORIES

MEAL 4 Time: _____	PROTEIN	CARBS	FATS	CALORIES

MEAL 5 Time: _____	PROTEIN	CARBS	FATS	CALORIES

DAILY TOTALS:				
UNDER / OVER TARGET:				

DATE: / /   DAY: M T W T F S S

HEALTH INVENTORY

TRAINING & IMPACT

Training day?:   ● HELL YEAH!   ● ACTIVE REST   ● DAY OFF
Intensity: ● HEAVY   ● AVERAGE   ● LIGHT

PERI-WORKOUT NUTRITION

Pre-workout:, intra- & post-workout nutrition / supplements:

MOOD & HUNGER

Hunger level?:   ● UNBEARABLE!   ● I CAN DEAL   ● WHAT HUNGER?
Overall mood:

CRAVINGS & TIME OF MONTH

Stage of menstrual cycle?:   ● MENSTRUAL   ● FOLLICULAR
Day: ● OVULATION   ● LUTEAL

Any cravings today?:

HYDRATION

Water intake: ● OVER TARGET!   ● ON TRACK   ● MUST DO BETTER
Glasses:

NOTES

DAILY FOOD LOG

MEAL 1	Time: _____	PROTEIN	CARBS	FATS	CALORIES

MEAL 2	Time: _____	PROTEIN	CARBS	FATS	CALORIES

MEAL 3	Time: _____	PROTEIN	CARBS	FATS	CALORIES

MEAL 4	Time: _____	PROTEIN	CARBS	FATS	CALORIES

MEAL 5	Time: _____	PROTEIN	CARBS	FATS	CALORIES

	PROTEIN	CARBS	FATS	CALORIES
DAILY TOTALS:				
UNDER / OVER TARGET:				

DATE: /   /   DAY: M T W T F S S

HEALTH INVENTORY

TRAINING & IMPACT

Training day?:   ● HELL YEAH!   ● ACTIVE REST   ● DAY OFF
Intensity: ● HEAVY   ● AVERAGE   ● LIGHT

PERI-WORKOUT NUTRITION

Pre-workout:, intra- & post-workout nutrition / supplements:

_____

_____

_____

MOOD & HUNGER

Hunger level?:   ● UNBEARABLE!   ● I CAN DEAL   ● WHAT HUNGER?
Overall mood: _____

CRAVINGS & TIME OF MONTH

Stage of menstrual cycle?:   ● MENSTRUAL   ● FOLLICULAR
Day: ● OVULATION   ● LUTEAL

Any cravings today?: _____

HYDRATION

Water intake: ● OVER TARGET!   ● ON TRACK   ● MUST DO BETTER
Glasses: _____

NOTES

_____

_____

DAILY FOOD LOG

MEAL 1 Time: _____	PROTEIN	CARBS	FATS	CALORIES

MEAL 2 Time: _____	PROTEIN	CARBS	FATS	CALORIES

MEAL 3 Time: _____	PROTEIN	CARBS	FATS	CALORIES

MEAL 4 Time: _____	PROTEIN	CARBS	FATS	CALORIES

MEAL 5 Time: _____	PROTEIN	CARBS	FATS	CALORIES

	PROTEIN	CARBS	FATS	CALORIES
DAILY TOTALS:				
UNDER / OVER TARGET:				

NOTES

MONTHLY CHECK-IN

DATE: /   /   DAY: M   T   W   T   F   S   S

Weight:

Body fat %:

Lean mass %:

Water %:

MEASUREMENTS

Neck:

Shoulders:

Chest / Bust:

Bicep (Left):   Bicep (Right):

Waist:

Hips:

Glutes:

Thigh (Left):   Thigh (Right):

Knee (Left):   Knee (Right):

Calf (Left):   Calf (Right):

NOTES

DATE: / /   DAY: M T W T F S S

HEALTH INVENTORY

TRAINING & IMPACT

Training day?:   ● HELL YEAH!   ● ACTIVE REST   ● DAY OFF

Intensity: ● HEAVY   ● AVERAGE   ● LIGHT

PERI-WORKOUT NUTRITION

Pre-workout:, intra- & post-workout nutrition / supplements:

MOOD & HUNGER

Hunger level?:   ● UNBEARABLE!   ● I CAN DEAL   ● WHAT HUNGER?

Overall mood:

CRAVINGS & TIME OF MONTH

Stage of menstrual cycle?:   ● MENSTRUAL   ● FOLLICULAR

Day: ● OVULATION   ● LUTEAL

Any cravings today?:

HYDRATION

Water intake: ● OVER TARGET!   ● ON TRACK   ● MUST DO BETTER

Glasses:

NOTES

DAILY FOOD LOG

MEAL 1　　Time: ____	PROTEIN	CARBS	FATS	CALORIES

MEAL 2　　Time: ____	PROTEIN	CARBS	FATS	CALORIES

MEAL 3　　Time: ____	PROTEIN	CARBS	FATS	CALORIES

MEAL 4　　Time: ____	PROTEIN	CARBS	FATS	CALORIES

MEAL 5　　Time: ____	PROTEIN	CARBS	FATS	CALORIES

	PROTEIN	CARBS	FATS	CALORIES
DAILY TOTALS:				
UNDER / OVER TARGET:				

DATE: / / DAY: M T W T F S S

HEALTH INVENTORY

TRAINING & IMPACT

Training day?: ● HELL YEAH! ● ACTIVE REST ● DAY OFF

Intensity: ● HEAVY ● AVERAGE ● LIGHT

PERI-WORKOUT NUTRITION

Pre-workout:, intra- & post-workout nutrition / supplements:

MOOD & HUNGER

Hunger level?: ● UNBEARABLE! ● I CAN DEAL ● WHAT HUNGER?

Overall mood:

CRAVINGS & TIME OF MONTH

Stage of menstrual cycle?: ● MENSTRUAL ● FOLLICULAR

Day: ● OVULATION ● LUTEAL

Any cravings today?:

HYDRATION

Water intake: ● OVER TARGET! ● ON TRACK ● MUST DO BETTER

Glasses:

NOTES

DAILY FOOD LOG

MEAL 1 Time: _____	PROTEIN	CARBS	FATS	CALORIES

MEAL 2 Time: _____	PROTEIN	CARBS	FATS	CALORIES

MEAL 3 Time: _____	PROTEIN	CARBS	FATS	CALORIES

MEAL 4 Time: _____	PROTEIN	CARBS	FATS	CALORIES

MEAL 5 Time: _____	PROTEIN	CARBS	FATS	CALORIES

	PROTEIN	CARBS	FATS	CALORIES
DAILY TOTALS:				
UNDER / OVER TARGET:				

DATE: / / DAY: M T W T F S S

HEALTH INVENTORY

TRAINING & IMPACT

Training day?: ● HELL YEAH! ● ACTIVE REST ● DAY OFF

Intensity: ● HEAVY ● AVERAGE ● LIGHT

PERI-WORKOUT NUTRITION

Pre-workout:, intra- & post-workout nutrition / supplements:

MOOD & HUNGER

Hunger level?: ● UNBEARABLE! ● I CAN DEAL ● WHAT HUNGER?

Overall mood:

CRAVINGS & TIME OF MONTH

Stage of menstrual cycle?: ● MENSTRUAL ● FOLLICULAR

Day: ● OVULATION ● LUTEAL

Any cravings today?:

HYDRATION

Water intake: ● OVER TARGET! ● ON TRACK ● MUST DO BETTER

Glasses:

NOTES

DAILY FOOD LOG

MEAL 1 Time: _____	PROTEIN	CARBS	FATS	CALORIES

MEAL 2 Time: _____	PROTEIN	CARBS	FATS	CALORIES

MEAL 3 Time: _____	PROTEIN	CARBS	FATS	CALORIES

MEAL 4 Time: _____	PROTEIN	CARBS	FATS	CALORIES

MEAL 5 Time: _____	PROTEIN	CARBS	FATS	CALORIES

DAILY TOTALS:				
UNDER / OVER TARGET:				

DATE: / /   DAY: M T W T F S S

HEALTH INVENTORY

TRAINING & IMPACT

Training day?:   ● HELL YEAH!   ● ACTIVE REST   ● DAY OFF
Intensity: ● HEAVY   ● AVERAGE   ● LIGHT

PERI-WORKOUT NUTRITION

Pre-workout:, intra- & post-workout nutrition / supplements:

MOOD & HUNGER

Hunger level?:   ● UNBEARABLE!   ● I CAN DEAL   ● WHAT HUNGER?
Overall mood:

CRAVINGS & TIME OF MONTH

Stage of menstrual cycle?:   ● MENSTRUAL   ● FOLLICULAR
                                    ● OVULATION   ● LUTEAL
Day:

Any cravings today?:

HYDRATION

Water intake: ● OVER TARGET!   ● ON TRACK   ● MUST DO BETTER
Glasses:

NOTES

DAILY FOOD LOG

MEAL 1	Time: _____	PROTEIN	CARBS	FATS	CALORIES

MEAL 2	Time: _____	PROTEIN	CARBS	FATS	CALORIES

MEAL 3	Time: _____	PROTEIN	CARBS	FATS	CALORIES

MEAL 4	Time: _____	PROTEIN	CARBS	FATS	CALORIES

MEAL 5	Time: _____	PROTEIN	CARBS	FATS	CALORIES

DAILY TOTALS:				
UNDER / OVER TARGET:				

DATE: / / DAY: M T W T F S S

HEALTH INVENTORY

TRAINING & IMPACT

Training day?: ● HELL YEAH! ● ACTIVE REST ● DAY OFF

Intensity: ● HEAVY ● AVERAGE ● LIGHT

PERI-WORKOUT NUTRITION

Pre-workout:, intra- & post-workout nutrition / supplements:

MOOD & HUNGER

Hunger level?: ● UNBEARABLE! ● I CAN DEAL ● WHAT HUNGER?

Overall mood:

CRAVINGS & TIME OF MONTH

Stage of menstrual cycle?: ● MENSTRUAL ● FOLLICULAR

Day: ● OVULATION ● LUTEAL

Any cravings today?:

HYDRATION

Water intake: ● OVER TARGET! ● ON TRACK ● MUST DO BETTER

Glasses:

NOTES

DAILY FOOD LOG

MEAL 1 Time: _____	PROTEIN	CARBS	FATS	CALORIES

MEAL 2 Time: _____	PROTEIN	CARBS	FATS	CALORIES

MEAL 3 Time: _____	PROTEIN	CARBS	FATS	CALORIES

MEAL 4 Time: _____	PROTEIN	CARBS	FATS	CALORIES

MEAL 5 Time: _____	PROTEIN	CARBS	FATS	CALORIES

	PROTEIN	CARBS	FATS	CALORIES
DAILY TOTALS:				
UNDER / OVER TARGET:				

DATE: / / DAY: M T W T F S S

HEALTH INVENTORY

TRAINING & IMPACT

Training day?: ● HELL YEAH! ● ACTIVE REST ● DAY OFF

Intensity: ● HEAVY ● AVERAGE ● LIGHT

PERI-WORKOUT NUTRITION

Pre-workout:, intra- & post-workout nutrition / supplements:

MOOD & HUNGER

Hunger level?: ● UNBEARABLE! ● I CAN DEAL ● WHAT HUNGER?

Overall mood:

CRAVINGS & TIME OF MONTH

Stage of menstrual cycle?: ● MENSTRUAL ● FOLLICULAR

Day: ● OVULATION ● LUTEAL

Any cravings today?:

HYDRATION

Water intake: ● OVER TARGET! ● ON TRACK ● MUST DO BETTER

Glasses:

NOTES

DAILY FOOD LOG

MEAL 1 Time: _____	PROTEIN	CARBS	FATS	CALORIES

MEAL 2 Time: _____	PROTEIN	CARBS	FATS	CALORIES

MEAL 3 Time: _____	PROTEIN	CARBS	FATS	CALORIES

MEAL 4 Time: _____	PROTEIN	CARBS	FATS	CALORIES

MEAL 5 Time: _____	PROTEIN	CARBS	FATS	CALORIES

DAILY TOTALS:				
UNDER / OVER TARGET:				

HEALTH INVENTORY

TRAINING & IMPACT

Training day?:   ● HELL YEAH!   ● ACTIVE REST   ● DAY OFF

Intensity: ● HEAVY   ● AVERAGE   ● LIGHT

PERI-WORKOUT NUTRITION

Pre-workout:, intra- & post-workout nutrition / supplements:

MOOD & HUNGER

Hunger level?:   ● UNBEARABLE!   ● I CAN DEAL   ● WHAT HUNGER?

Overall mood:

CRAVINGS & TIME OF MONTH

Stage of menstrual cycle?:   ● MENSTRUAL   ● FOLLICULAR

Day: ● OVULATION   ● LUTEAL

Any cravings today?:

HYDRATION

Water intake: ● OVER TARGET!   ● ON TRACK   ● MUST DO BETTER

Glasses:

NOTES

DAILY FOOD LOG

MEAL 1 Time: _____	PROTEIN	CARBS	FATS	CALORIES

MEAL 2 Time: _____	PROTEIN	CARBS	FATS	CALORIES

MEAL 3 Time: _____	PROTEIN	CARBS	FATS	CALORIES

MEAL 4 Time: _____	PROTEIN	CARBS	FATS	CALORIES

MEAL 5 Time: _____	PROTEIN	CARBS	FATS	CALORIES

	PROTEIN	CARBS	FATS	CALORIES
DAILY TOTALS:				
UNDER / OVER TARGET:				

DATE: / / DAY: M T W T F S S

HEALTH INVENTORY

TRAINING & IMPACT

Training day?:   ● HELL YEAH!   ● ACTIVE REST   ● DAY OFF

Intensity: ● HEAVY   ● AVERAGE   ● LIGHT

PERI-WORKOUT NUTRITION

Pre-workout:, intra- & post-workout nutrition / supplements:

MOOD & HUNGER

Hunger level?:   ● UNBEARABLE!   ● I CAN DEAL   ● WHAT HUNGER?

Overall mood:

CRAVINGS & TIME OF MONTH

Stage of menstrual cycle?:   ● MENSTRUAL   ● FOLLICULAR

Day: ● OVULATION   ● LUTEAL

Any cravings today?:

HYDRATION

Water intake: ● OVER TARGET!   ● ON TRACK   ● MUST DO BETTER

Glasses:

NOTES

DAILY FOOD LOG

MEAL 1 Time: _____	PROTEIN	CARBS	FATS	CALORIES

MEAL 2 Time: _____	PROTEIN	CARBS	FATS	CALORIES

MEAL 3 Time: _____	PROTEIN	CARBS	FATS	CALORIES

MEAL 4 Time: _____	PROTEIN	CARBS	FATS	CALORIES

MEAL 5 Time: _____	PROTEIN	CARBS	FATS	CALORIES

DAILY TOTALS:				
UNDER / OVER TARGET:				

DATE: /   /   DAY: M T W T F S S

HEALTH INVENTORY

TRAINING & IMPACT

Training day?:   ● HELL YEAH!   ● ACTIVE REST   ● DAY OFF

Intensity: ● HEAVY   ● AVERAGE   ● LIGHT

PERI-WORKOUT NUTRITION

Pre-workout:, intra- & post-workout nutrition / supplements:

....

....

....

MOOD & HUNGER

Hunger level?:   ● UNBEARABLE!   ● I CAN DEAL   ● WHAT HUNGER?

Overall mood: ....

CRAVINGS & TIME OF MONTH

Stage of menstrual cycle?:   ● MENSTRUAL   ● FOLLICULAR

Day: ● OVULATION   ● LUTEAL

Any cravings today?: ....

HYDRATION

Water intake: ● OVER TARGET!   ● ON TRACK   ● MUST DO BETTER

Glasses: ....

NOTES

....

....

DAILY FOOD LOG

MEAL 1	Time: _____	PROTEIN	CARBS	FATS	CALORIES

MEAL 2	Time: _____	PROTEIN	CARBS	FATS	CALORIES

MEAL 3	Time: _____	PROTEIN	CARBS	FATS	CALORIES

MEAL 4	Time: _____	PROTEIN	CARBS	FATS	CALORIES

MEAL 5	Time: _____	PROTEIN	CARBS	FATS	CALORIES

	PROTEIN	CARBS	FATS	CALORIES
DAILY TOTALS:				
UNDER / OVER TARGET:				

DATE: / / DAY: M T W T F S S

HEALTH INVENTORY

TRAINING & IMPACT

Training day?: ● HELL YEAH! ● ACTIVE REST ● DAY OFF

Intensity: ● HEAVY ● AVERAGE ● LIGHT

PERI-WORKOUT NUTRITION

Pre-workout:, intra- & post-workout nutrition / supplements:

MOOD & HUNGER

Hunger level?: ● UNBEARABLE! ● I CAN DEAL ● WHAT HUNGER?

Overall mood:

CRAVINGS & TIME OF MONTH

Stage of menstrual cycle?: ● MENSTRUAL ● FOLLICULAR

Day: ● OVULATION ● LUTEAL

Any cravings today?:

HYDRATION

Water intake: ● OVER TARGET! ● ON TRACK ● MUST DO BETTER

Glasses:

NOTES

DAILY FOOD LOG

MEAL 1 Time: _____	PROTEIN	CARBS	FATS	CALORIES

MEAL 2 Time: _____	PROTEIN	CARBS	FATS	CALORIES

MEAL 3 Time: _____	PROTEIN	CARBS	FATS	CALORIES

MEAL 4 Time: _____	PROTEIN	CARBS	FATS	CALORIES

MEAL 5 Time: _____	PROTEIN	CARBS	FATS	CALORIES

DAILY TOTALS:				
UNDER / OVER TARGET:				

DATE: / /   DAY: M T W T F S S

HEALTH INVENTORY

TRAINING & IMPACT

Training day?:   ● HELL YEAH!   ● ACTIVE REST   ● DAY OFF

Intensity: ● HEAVY   ● AVERAGE   ● LIGHT

PERI-WORKOUT NUTRITION

Pre-workout:, intra- & post-workout nutrition / supplements:

....

....

....

MOOD & HUNGER

Hunger level?:   ● UNBEARABLE!   ● I CAN DEAL   ● WHAT HUNGER?

Overall mood: ....

CRAVINGS & TIME OF MONTH

Stage of menstrual cycle?:   ● MENSTRUAL   ● FOLLICULAR

Day: ● OVULATION   ● LUTEAL

Any cravings today?: ....

HYDRATION

Water intake: ● OVER TARGET!   ● ON TRACK   ● MUST DO BETTER

Glasses: ....

NOTES ....

....

DAILY FOOD LOG

MEAL 1 Time: ____	PROTEIN	CARBS	FATS	CALORIES

MEAL 2 Time: ____	PROTEIN	CARBS	FATS	CALORIES

MEAL 3 Time: ____	PROTEIN	CARBS	FATS	CALORIES

MEAL 4 Time: ____	PROTEIN	CARBS	FATS	CALORIES

MEAL 5 Time: ____	PROTEIN	CARBS	FATS	CALORIES

DAILY TOTALS:				
UNDER / OVER TARGET:				

HEALTH INVENTORY

TRAINING & IMPACT

Training day?:   ● HELL YEAH!   ● ACTIVE REST   ● DAY OFF

Intensity: ● HEAVY   ● AVERAGE   ● LIGHT

PERI-WORKOUT NUTRITION

Pre-workout:, intra- & post-workout nutrition / supplements:

MOOD & HUNGER

Hunger level?:   ● UNBEARABLE!   ● I CAN DEAL   ● WHAT HUNGER?

Overall mood:

CRAVINGS & TIME OF MONTH

Stage of menstrual cycle?:   ● MENSTRUAL   ● FOLLICULAR

Day: ● OVULATION   ● LUTEAL

Any cravings today?:

HYDRATION

Water intake: ● OVER TARGET!   ● ON TRACK   ● MUST DO BETTER

Glasses:

NOTES

DAILY FOOD LOG

MEAL 1 Time: _____	PROTEIN	CARBS	FATS	CALORIES

MEAL 2 Time: _____	PROTEIN	CARBS	FATS	CALORIES

MEAL 3 Time: _____	PROTEIN	CARBS	FATS	CALORIES

MEAL 4 Time: _____	PROTEIN	CARBS	FATS	CALORIES

MEAL 5 Time: _____	PROTEIN	CARBS	FATS	CALORIES

DAILY TOTALS:				
UNDER / OVER TARGET:				

HEALTH INVENTORY

TRAINING & IMPACT

Training day?:   ● HELL YEAH!   ● ACTIVE REST   ● DAY OFF

Intensity: ● HEAVY   ● AVERAGE   ● LIGHT

PERI-WORKOUT NUTRITION

Pre-workout:, intra- & post-workout nutrition / supplements:

MOOD & HUNGER

Hunger level?:   ● UNBEARABLE!   ● I CAN DEAL   ● WHAT HUNGER?

Overall mood:

CRAVINGS & TIME OF MONTH

Stage of menstrual cycle?:   ● MENSTRUAL   ● FOLLICULAR

Day: ● OVULATION   ● LUTEAL

Any cravings today?:

HYDRATION

Water intake: ● OVER TARGET!   ● ON TRACK   ● MUST DO BETTER

Glasses:

NOTES

DAILY FOOD LOG

MEAL 1 Time: _____	PROTEIN	CARBS	FATS	CALORIES

MEAL 2 Time: _____	PROTEIN	CARBS	FATS	CALORIES

MEAL 3 Time: _____	PROTEIN	CARBS	FATS	CALORIES

MEAL 4 Time: _____	PROTEIN	CARBS	FATS	CALORIES

MEAL 5 Time: _____	PROTEIN	CARBS	FATS	CALORIES

	PROTEIN	CARBS	FATS	CALORIES
DAILY TOTALS:				
UNDER / OVER TARGET:				

DATE: /   /   DAY: M T W T F S S

HEALTH INVENTORY

TRAINING & IMPACT

Training day?:   ● HELL YEAH!   ● ACTIVE REST   ● DAY OFF

Intensity: ● HEAVY   ● AVERAGE   ● LIGHT

PERI-WORKOUT NUTRITION

Pre-workout:, intra- & post-workout nutrition / supplements:

MOOD & HUNGER

Hunger level?:   ● UNBEARABLE!   ● I CAN DEAL   ● WHAT HUNGER?

Overall mood:

CRAVINGS & TIME OF MONTH

Stage of menstrual cycle?:   ● MENSTRUAL   ● FOLLICULAR

Day: ● OVULATION   ● LUTEAL

Any cravings today?:

HYDRATION

Water intake: ● OVER TARGET!   ● ON TRACK   ● MUST DO BETTER

Glasses:

NOTES

DAILY FOOD LOG

MEAL 1 Time: _____	PROTEIN	CARBS	FATS	CALORIES

MEAL 2 Time: _____	PROTEIN	CARBS	FATS	CALORIES

MEAL 3 Time: _____	PROTEIN	CARBS	FATS	CALORIES

MEAL 4 Time: _____	PROTEIN	CARBS	FATS	CALORIES

MEAL 5 Time: _____	PROTEIN	CARBS	FATS	CALORIES

DAILY TOTALS:				
UNDER / OVER TARGET:				

DATE: /   /   DAY: M   T   W   T   F   S   S

HEALTH INVENTORY

TRAINING & IMPACT

Training day?:   ⬤ HELL YEAH!   ⬤ ACTIVE REST   ⬤ DAY OFF

Intensity: ⬤ HEAVY   ⬤ AVERAGE   ⬤ LIGHT

PERI-WORKOUT NUTRITION

Pre-workout:, intra- & post-workout nutrition / supplements:

MOOD & HUNGER

Hunger level?:   ⬤ UNBEARABLE!   ⬤ I CAN DEAL   ⬤ WHAT HUNGER?

Overall mood:

CRAVINGS & TIME OF MONTH

Stage of menstrual cycle?:   ⬤ MENSTRUAL   ⬤ FOLLICULAR

Day: ⬤ OVULATION   ⬤ LUTEAL

Any cravings today?:

HYDRATION

Water intake: ⬤ OVER TARGET!   ⬤ ON TRACK   ⬤ MUST DO BETTER

Glasses:

NOTES

DAILY FOOD LOG

MEAL 1 Time: _____	PROTEIN	CARBS	FATS	CALORIES

MEAL 2 Time: _____	PROTEIN	CARBS	FATS	CALORIES

MEAL 3 Time: _____	PROTEIN	CARBS	FATS	CALORIES

MEAL 4 Time: _____	PROTEIN	CARBS	FATS	CALORIES

MEAL 5 Time: _____	PROTEIN	CARBS	FATS	CALORIES

	PROTEIN	CARBS	FATS	CALORIES
DAILY TOTALS:				
UNDER / OVER TARGET:				

DATE: / /   DAY: M T W T F S S

HEALTH INVENTORY

TRAINING & IMPACT

Training day?:   ⬤ HELL YEAH!   ⬤ ACTIVE REST   ⬤ DAY OFF

Intensity: ⬤ HEAVY   ⬤ AVERAGE   ⬤ LIGHT

PERI-WORKOUT NUTRITION

Pre-workout:, intra- & post-workout nutrition / supplements:

MOOD & HUNGER

Hunger level?:   ⬤ UNBEARABLE!   ⬤ I CAN DEAL   ⬤ WHAT HUNGER?

Overall mood:

CRAVINGS & TIME OF MONTH

Stage of menstrual cycle?:   ⬤ MENSTRUAL   ⬤ FOLLICULAR

Day: ⬤ OVULATION   ⬤ LUTEAL

Any cravings today?:

HYDRATION

Water intake: ⬤ OVER TARGET!   ⬤ ON TRACK   ⬤ MUST DO BETTER

Glasses:

NOTES

DAILY FOOD LOG

MEAL 1 Time: _____	PROTEIN	CARBS	FATS	CALORIES

MEAL 2 Time: _____	PROTEIN	CARBS	FATS	CALORIES

MEAL 3 Time: _____	PROTEIN	CARBS	FATS	CALORIES

MEAL 4 Time: _____	PROTEIN	CARBS	FATS	CALORIES

MEAL 5 Time: _____	PROTEIN	CARBS	FATS	CALORIES

DAILY TOTALS:				
UNDER / OVER TARGET:				

DATE: / /   DAY: M T W T F S S

HEALTH INVENTORY

TRAINING & IMPACT

Training day?:   ● HELL YEAH!   ● ACTIVE REST   ● DAY OFF

Intensity: ● HEAVY   ● AVERAGE   ● LIGHT

PERI-WORKOUT NUTRITION

Pre-workout:, intra- & post-workout nutrition / supplements:

MOOD & HUNGER

Hunger level?:   ● UNBEARABLE!   ● I CAN DEAL   ● WHAT HUNGER?

Overall mood:

CRAVINGS & TIME OF MONTH

Stage of menstrual cycle?:   ● MENSTRUAL   ● FOLLICULAR

Day: ● OVULATION   ● LUTEAL

Any cravings today?:

HYDRATION

Water intake: ● OVER TARGET!   ● ON TRACK   ● MUST DO BETTER

Glasses:

NOTES

DAILY FOOD LOG

MEAL 1 Time: _____	PROTEIN	CARBS	FATS	CALORIES

MEAL 2 Time: _____	PROTEIN	CARBS	FATS	CALORIES

MEAL 3 Time: _____	PROTEIN	CARBS	FATS	CALORIES

MEAL 4 Time: _____	PROTEIN	CARBS	FATS	CALORIES

MEAL 5 Time: _____	PROTEIN	CARBS	FATS	CALORIES

DAILY TOTALS:				
UNDER / OVER TARGET:				

DATE: / /   DAY: M T W T F S S

HEALTH INVENTORY

TRAINING & IMPACT

Training day?:   ● HELL YEAH!   ● ACTIVE REST   ● DAY OFF

Intensity: ● HEAVY   ● AVERAGE   ● LIGHT

PERI-WORKOUT NUTRITION

Pre-workout:, intra- & post-workout nutrition / supplements:

MOOD & HUNGER

Hunger level?:   ● UNBEARABLE!   ● I CAN DEAL   ● WHAT HUNGER?

Overall mood:

CRAVINGS & TIME OF MONTH

Stage of menstrual cycle?:   ● MENSTRUAL   ● FOLLICULAR

Day: ● OVULATION   ● LUTEAL

Any cravings today?:

HYDRATION

Water intake: ● OVER TARGET!   ● ON TRACK   ● MUST DO BETTER

Glasses:

NOTES

DAILY FOOD LOG

MEAL 1	Time: _____	PROTEIN	CARBS	FATS	CALORIES

MEAL 2	Time: _____	PROTEIN	CARBS	FATS	CALORIES

MEAL 3	Time: _____	PROTEIN	CARBS	FATS	CALORIES

MEAL 4	Time: _____	PROTEIN	CARBS	FATS	CALORIES

MEAL 5	Time: _____	PROTEIN	CARBS	FATS	CALORIES

DAILY TOTALS:				
UNDER / OVER TARGET:				

DATE: /   /   DAY: M   T   W   T   F   S   S

HEALTH INVENTORY

TRAINING & IMPACT

Training day?:   ● HELL YEAH!   ● ACTIVE REST   ● DAY OFF

Intensity: ● HEAVY   ● AVERAGE   ● LIGHT

PERI-WORKOUT NUTRITION

Pre-workout:, intra- & post-workout nutrition / supplements:

MOOD & HUNGER

Hunger level?:   ● UNBEARABLE!   ● I CAN DEAL   ● WHAT HUNGER?

Overall mood:

CRAVINGS & TIME OF MONTH

Stage of menstrual cycle?:   ● MENSTRUAL   ● FOLLICULAR

Day: ● OVULATION   ● LUTEAL

Any cravings today?:

HYDRATION

Water intake: ● OVER TARGET!   ● ON TRACK   ● MUST DO BETTER

Glasses:

NOTES

DAILY FOOD LOG

MEAL 1 Time: _____	PROTEIN	CARBS	FATS	CALORIES

MEAL 2 Time: _____	PROTEIN	CARBS	FATS	CALORIES

MEAL 3 Time: _____	PROTEIN	CARBS	FATS	CALORIES

MEAL 4 Time: _____	PROTEIN	CARBS	FATS	CALORIES

MEAL 5 Time: _____	PROTEIN	CARBS	FATS	CALORIES

DAILY TOTALS:				
UNDER / OVER TARGET:				

DATE: /   /   DAY: M T W T F S S

HEALTH INVENTORY

TRAINING & IMPACT

Training day?:   ● HELL YEAH!   ● ACTIVE REST   ● DAY OFF

Intensity: ● HEAVY   ● AVERAGE   ● LIGHT

PERI-WORKOUT NUTRITION

Pre-workout:, intra- & post-workout nutrition / supplements:

MOOD & HUNGER

Hunger level?:   ● UNBEARABLE!   ● I CAN DEAL   ● WHAT HUNGER?

Overall mood:

CRAVINGS & TIME OF MONTH

Stage of menstrual cycle?:   ● MENSTRUAL   ● FOLLICULAR

Day: ● OVULATION   ● LUTEAL

Any cravings today?:

HYDRATION

Water intake: ● OVER TARGET!   ● ON TRACK   ● MUST DO BETTER

Glasses:

NOTES

DAILY FOOD LOG

MEAL 1 Time: _____	PROTEIN	CARBS	FATS	CALORIES

MEAL 2 Time: _____	PROTEIN	CARBS	FATS	CALORIES

MEAL 3 Time: _____	PROTEIN	CARBS	FATS	CALORIES

MEAL 4 Time: _____	PROTEIN	CARBS	FATS	CALORIES

MEAL 5 Time: _____	PROTEIN	CARBS	FATS	CALORIES

DAILY TOTALS:				
UNDER / OVER TARGET:				

DATE: / / DAY: M T W T F S S

HEALTH INVENTORY

TRAINING & IMPACT

Training day?: ● HELL YEAH! ● ACTIVE REST ● DAY OFF

Intensity: ● HEAVY ● AVERAGE ● LIGHT

PERI-WORKOUT NUTRITION

Pre-workout:, intra- & post-workout nutrition / supplements:

MOOD & HUNGER

Hunger level?: ● UNBEARABLE! ● I CAN DEAL ● WHAT HUNGER?

Overall mood:

CRAVINGS & TIME OF MONTH

Stage of menstrual cycle?: ● MENSTRUAL ● FOLLICULAR

Day: ● OVULATION ● LUTEAL

Any cravings today?:

HYDRATION

Water intake: ● OVER TARGET! ● ON TRACK ● MUST DO BETTER

Glasses:

NOTES

DAILY FOOD LOG

MEAL 1 Time: _____	PROTEIN	CARBS	FATS	CALORIES

MEAL 2 Time: _____	PROTEIN	CARBS	FATS	CALORIES

MEAL 3 Time: _____	PROTEIN	CARBS	FATS	CALORIES

MEAL 4 Time: _____	PROTEIN	CARBS	FATS	CALORIES

MEAL 5 Time: _____	PROTEIN	CARBS	FATS	CALORIES

	PROTEIN	CARBS	FATS	CALORIES
DAILY TOTALS:				
UNDER / OVER TARGET:				

DATE: / / DAY: M T W T F S S

HEALTH INVENTORY

TRAINING & IMPACT

Training day?: ● HELL YEAH! ● ACTIVE REST ● DAY OFF

Intensity: ● HEAVY ● AVERAGE ● LIGHT

PERI-WORKOUT NUTRITION

Pre-workout:, intra- & post-workout nutrition / supplements:

MOOD & HUNGER

Hunger level?: ● UNBEARABLE! ● I CAN DEAL ● WHAT HUNGER?

Overall mood:

CRAVINGS & TIME OF MONTH

Stage of menstrual cycle?: ● MENSTRUAL ● FOLLICULAR

Day: ● OVULATION ● LUTEAL

Any cravings today?:

HYDRATION

Water intake: ● OVER TARGET! ● ON TRACK ● MUST DO BETTER

Glasses:

NOTES

DAILY FOOD LOG

MEAL 1 Time: _____	PROTEIN	CARBS	FATS	CALORIES

MEAL 2 Time: _____	PROTEIN	CARBS	FATS	CALORIES

MEAL 3 Time: _____	PROTEIN	CARBS	FATS	CALORIES

MEAL 4 Time: _____	PROTEIN	CARBS	FATS	CALORIES

MEAL 5 Time: _____	PROTEIN	CARBS	FATS	CALORIES

DAILY TOTALS:				
UNDER / OVER TARGET:				

DATE: /   /   DAY: M   T   W   T   F   S   S

HEALTH INVENTORY

TRAINING & IMPACT

Training day?:   ● HELL YEAH!   ● ACTIVE REST   ● DAY OFF

Intensity: ● HEAVY   ● AVERAGE   ● LIGHT

PERI-WORKOUT NUTRITION

Pre-workout:, intra- & post-workout nutrition / supplements:

MOOD & HUNGER

Hunger level?:   ● UNBEARABLE!   ● I CAN DEAL   ● WHAT HUNGER?

Overall mood:

CRAVINGS & TIME OF MONTH

Stage of menstrual cycle?:   ● MENSTRUAL   ● FOLLICULAR

Day: ● OVULATION   ● LUTEAL

Any cravings today?:

HYDRATION

Water intake: ● OVER TARGET!   ● ON TRACK   ● MUST DO BETTER

Glasses:

NOTES

DAILY FOOD LOG

MEAL 1 Time: _____	PROTEIN	CARBS	FATS	CALORIES

MEAL 2 Time: _____	PROTEIN	CARBS	FATS	CALORIES

MEAL 3 Time: _____	PROTEIN	CARBS	FATS	CALORIES

MEAL 4 Time: _____	PROTEIN	CARBS	FATS	CALORIES

MEAL 5 Time: _____	PROTEIN	CARBS	FATS	CALORIES

	PROTEIN	CARBS	FATS	CALORIES
DAILY TOTALS:				
UNDER / OVER TARGET:				

DATE: /   /   DAY: M T W T F S S

HEALTH INVENTORY

TRAINING & IMPACT

Training day?:   ● HELL YEAH!   ● ACTIVE REST   ● DAY OFF

Intensity: ● HEAVY   ● AVERAGE   ● LIGHT

PERI-WORKOUT NUTRITION

Pre-workout:, intra- & post-workout nutrition / supplements:

MOOD & HUNGER

Hunger level?:   ● UNBEARABLE!   ● I CAN DEAL   ● WHAT HUNGER?

Overall mood:

CRAVINGS & TIME OF MONTH

Stage of menstrual cycle?:   ● MENSTRUAL   ● FOLLICULAR

Day: ● OVULATION   ● LUTEAL

Any cravings today?:

HYDRATION

Water intake: ● OVER TARGET!   ● ON TRACK   ● MUST DO BETTER

Glasses:

NOTES

DAILY FOOD LOG

MEAL 1 Time: ____	PROTEIN	CARBS	FATS	CALORIES

MEAL 2 Time: ____	PROTEIN	CARBS	FATS	CALORIES

MEAL 3 Time: ____	PROTEIN	CARBS	FATS	CALORIES

MEAL 4 Time: ____	PROTEIN	CARBS	FATS	CALORIES

MEAL 5 Time: ____	PROTEIN	CARBS	FATS	CALORIES

	PROTEIN	CARBS	FATS	CALORIES
DAILY TOTALS:				
UNDER / OVER TARGET:				

DATE: /   /   DAY: M T W T F S S

HEALTH INVENTORY

TRAINING & IMPACT

Training day?:   ● HELL YEAH!   ● ACTIVE REST   ● DAY OFF

Intensity: ● HEAVY   ● AVERAGE   ● LIGHT

PERI-WORKOUT NUTRITION

Pre-workout:, intra- & post-workout nutrition / supplements:

MOOD & HUNGER

Hunger level?:   ● UNBEARABLE!   ● I CAN DEAL   ● WHAT HUNGER?

Overall mood:

CRAVINGS & TIME OF MONTH

Stage of menstrual cycle?:   ● MENSTRUAL   ● FOLLICULAR

Day: ● OVULATION   ● LUTEAL

Any cravings today?:

HYDRATION

Water intake: ● OVER TARGET!   ● ON TRACK   ● MUST DO BETTER

Glasses:

NOTES

DAILY FOOD LOG

MEAL 1 Time: _____	PROTEIN	CARBS	FATS	CALORIES

MEAL 2 Time: _____	PROTEIN	CARBS	FATS	CALORIES

MEAL 3 Time: _____	PROTEIN	CARBS	FATS	CALORIES

MEAL 4 Time: _____	PROTEIN	CARBS	FATS	CALORIES

MEAL 5 Time: _____	PROTEIN	CARBS	FATS	CALORIES

	PROTEIN	CARBS	FATS	CALORIES
DAILY TOTALS:				
UNDER / OVER TARGET:				

DATE: /   /   DAY: M   T   W   T   F   S   S

HEALTH INVENTORY

TRAINING & IMPACT

Training day?:   ● HELL YEAH!   ● ACTIVE REST   ● DAY OFF

Intensity: ● HEAVY   ● AVERAGE   ● LIGHT

PERI-WORKOUT NUTRITION

Pre-workout:, intra- & post-workout nutrition / supplements:

MOOD & HUNGER

Hunger level?:   ● UNBEARABLE!   ● I CAN DEAL   ● WHAT HUNGER?

Overall mood:

CRAVINGS & TIME OF MONTH

Stage of menstrual cycle?:   ● MENSTRUAL   ● FOLLICULAR

Day: ● OVULATION   ● LUTEAL

Any cravings today?:

HYDRATION

Water intake: ● OVER TARGET!   ● ON TRACK   ● MUST DO BETTER

Glasses:

NOTES

DAILY FOOD LOG

MEAL 1 Time: _____	PROTEIN	CARBS	FATS	CALORIES

MEAL 2 Time: _____	PROTEIN	CARBS	FATS	CALORIES

MEAL 3 Time: _____	PROTEIN	CARBS	FATS	CALORIES

MEAL 4 Time: _____	PROTEIN	CARBS	FATS	CALORIES

MEAL 5 Time: _____	PROTEIN	CARBS	FATS	CALORIES

DAILY TOTALS:				
UNDER / OVER TARGET:				

DATE: / / DAY: M T W T F S S

HEALTH INVENTORY

TRAINING & IMPACT

Training day?: ● HELL YEAH! ● ACTIVE REST ● DAY OFF
Intensity: ● HEAVY ● AVERAGE ● LIGHT

PERI-WORKOUT NUTRITION

Pre-workout:, intra- & post-workout nutrition / supplements:

MOOD & HUNGER

Hunger level?: ● UNBEARABLE! ● I CAN DEAL ● WHAT HUNGER?
Overall mood:

CRAVINGS & TIME OF MONTH

Stage of menstrual cycle?: ● MENSTRUAL ● FOLLICULAR
Day: ● OVULATION ● LUTEAL

Any cravings today?:

HYDRATION

Water intake: ● OVER TARGET! ● ON TRACK ● MUST DO BETTER
Glasses:

NOTES

DAILY FOOD LOG

MEAL 1	Time: _____	PROTEIN	CARBS	FATS	CALORIES

MEAL 2	Time: _____	PROTEIN	CARBS	FATS	CALORIES

MEAL 3	Time: _____	PROTEIN	CARBS	FATS	CALORIES

MEAL 4	Time: _____	PROTEIN	CARBS	FATS	CALORIES

MEAL 5	Time: _____	PROTEIN	CARBS	FATS	CALORIES

	PROTEIN	CARBS	FATS	CALORIES
DAILY TOTALS:				
UNDER / OVER TARGET:				

DATE: /   /   DAY: M   T   W   T   F   S   S

HEALTH INVENTORY

TRAINING & IMPACT

Training day?:   ⬤ HELL YEAH!   ⬤ ACTIVE REST   ⬤ DAY OFF

Intensity: ⬤ HEAVY   ⬤ AVERAGE   ⬤ LIGHT

PERI-WORKOUT NUTRITION

Pre-workout:, intra- & post-workout nutrition / supplements:

MOOD & HUNGER

Hunger level?:   ⬤ UNBEARABLE!   ⬤ I CAN DEAL   ⬤ WHAT HUNGER?

Overall mood:

CRAVINGS & TIME OF MONTH

Stage of menstrual cycle?:   ⬤ MENSTRUAL   ⬤ FOLLICULAR

Day: ⬤ OVULATION   ⬤ LUTEAL

Any cravings today?:

HYDRATION

Water intake: ⬤ OVER TARGET!   ⬤ ON TRACK   ⬤ MUST DO BETTER

Glasses:

NOTES

DAILY FOOD LOG

MEAL 1 Time: _____	PROTEIN	CARBS	FATS	CALORIES

MEAL 2 Time: _____	PROTEIN	CARBS	FATS	CALORIES

MEAL 3 Time: _____	PROTEIN	CARBS	FATS	CALORIES

MEAL 4 Time: _____	PROTEIN	CARBS	FATS	CALORIES

MEAL 5 Time: _____	PROTEIN	CARBS	FATS	CALORIES

DAILY TOTALS:				
UNDER / OVER TARGET:				

DATE: / /   DAY: M T W T F S S

HEALTH INVENTORY

TRAINING & IMPACT

Training day?: ● HELL YEAH!   ● ACTIVE REST   ● DAY OFF

Intensity: ● HEAVY   ● AVERAGE   ● LIGHT

PERI-WORKOUT NUTRITION

Pre-workout:, intra- & post-workout nutrition / supplements:

MOOD & HUNGER

Hunger level?: ● UNBEARABLE!   ● I CAN DEAL   ● WHAT HUNGER?

Overall mood:

CRAVINGS & TIME OF MONTH

Stage of menstrual cycle?:   ● MENSTRUAL   ● FOLLICULAR

Day: ● OVULATION   ● LUTEAL

Any cravings today?:

HYDRATION

Water intake: ● OVER TARGET!   ● ON TRACK   ● MUST DO BETTER

Glasses:

NOTES

DAILY FOOD LOG

MEAL 1 Time: _____	PROTEIN	CARBS	FATS	CALORIES

MEAL 2 Time: _____	PROTEIN	CARBS	FATS	CALORIES

MEAL 3 Time: _____	PROTEIN	CARBS	FATS	CALORIES

MEAL 4 Time: _____	PROTEIN	CARBS	FATS	CALORIES

MEAL 5 Time: _____	PROTEIN	CARBS	FATS	CALORIES

DAILY TOTALS:				
UNDER / OVER TARGET:				

DATE: / / DAY: M T W T F S S

HEALTH INVENTORY

TRAINING & IMPACT

Training day?:   ● HELL YEAH!   ● ACTIVE REST   ● DAY OFF

Intensity: ● HEAVY   ● AVERAGE   ● LIGHT

PERI-WORKOUT NUTRITION

Pre-workout:, intra- & post-workout nutrition / supplements:

MOOD & HUNGER

Hunger level?:   ● UNBEARABLE!   ● I CAN DEAL   ● WHAT HUNGER?

Overall mood:

CRAVINGS & TIME OF MONTH

Stage of menstrual cycle?:   ● MENSTRUAL   ● FOLLICULAR

Day: ● OVULATION   ● LUTEAL

Any cravings today?:

HYDRATION

Water intake: ● OVER TARGET!   ● ON TRACK   ● MUST DO BETTER

Glasses:

NOTES

DAILY FOOD LOG

MEAL 1 Time: _____	PROTEIN	CARBS	FATS	CALORIES

MEAL 2 Time: _____	PROTEIN	CARBS	FATS	CALORIES

MEAL 3 Time: _____	PROTEIN	CARBS	FATS	CALORIES

MEAL 4 Time: _____	PROTEIN	CARBS	FATS	CALORIES

MEAL 5 Time: _____	PROTEIN	CARBS	FATS	CALORIES

DAILY TOTALS:				
UNDER / OVER TARGET:				

NOTES

FINAL CHECK-IN

DATE: /   /   DAY: M   T   W   T   F   S   S

Weight:

Body fat %:

Lean mass %:

Water %:

MEASUREMENTS

Neck:

Shoulders:

Chest / Bust:

Bicep (Left):   Bicep (Right):

Waist:

Hips:

Glutes:

Thigh (Left):   Thigh (Right):

Knee (Left):   Knee (Right):

Calf (Left):   Calf (Right):

NOTES

MOTIVATION RE-CAP

Was I consistently motivated during this period?
What helped me to achieve my goals? Did anything hinder my progress?

GOALS RE-CAP

DAILY MACRONUTRIENT TARGETS

Was I able to consistently stick to my macro targets? If not, why?

NUTRITION GOALS

Goal 1:

Achieved: Y / N   If not, why?

Goal 2:

Achieved: Y / N   If not, why?

Goal 3:

Achieved: Y / N   If not, why?

HEALTHY LIVING GOALS

Goal 1:

Achieved: Y / N   If not, why?

Goal 2:

Achieved: Y / N   If not, why?

PHYSIQUE GOALS

Goal 1:

Achieved: Y / N   If not, why?

Goal 2:

Achieved: Y / N   If not, why?

NOTES

NOTES

NOTES

NOTES

Manufactured by Amazon.ca
Bolton, ON